CHINESE FACE READING

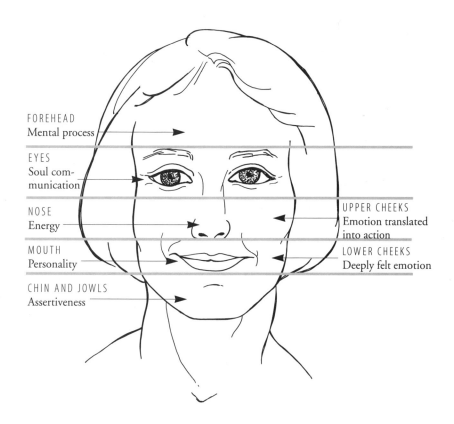

FOREHEAD
Mental process

EYES
Soul com-
munication

NOSE
Energy

MOUTH
Personality

CHIN AND JOWLS
Assertiveness

UPPER CHEEKS
Emotion translated
into action

LOWER CHEEKS
Deeply felt emotion

ACUPRESSURE POINTS

The stimulation of these points brings in vitality to improve skin tone and replaces the emotionally set face with an open countenance of well-being.

FOREHEAD POINTS 1
Affect mental clarity and improve blood circulation to the entire face.

EYEBROW POINT 2
Puts joy in residence on the face.

EYE POINTS 3
Open up sparkle in the eyes.

NOSE POINT 5
Energizes face.

CHEEK POINTS 4
Clear old, long-held emotions out of face.

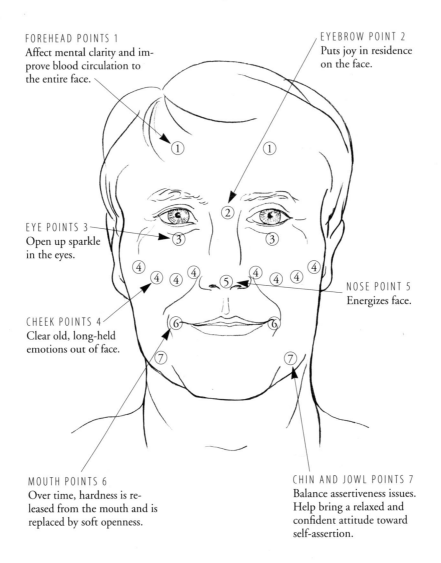

MOUTH POINTS 6
Over time, hardness is released from the mouth and is replaced by soft openness.

CHIN AND JOWL POINTS 7
Balance assertiveness issues. Help bring a relaxed and confident attitude toward self-assertion.

Timeless Face

Timeless Face

Thirty Days to a Younger You

Through Face Reading,

Acupressure, and Toning

Ellae Elinwood

St. Martin's Griffin
New York

Illustrations by Helen Redman
Photographs by Marilyn Davies and Robert Frost
Makeup by Roberto Guimaraes
Skin care by Epicuren Discovery

Design by Donna Sinisgalli

LIBRARY OF CONGRESS CATALOGING-IN-PUBLICATION DATA
Elinwood, Ellae.
    Timeless Face: thirty days to a younger you through face reading, acupressure, and toning / Ellae Elinwood.—1st [Griffin Trade pbk.] ed.
        p. cm.
    ISBN 0-312-19529-X
    1. Beauty, Personal. 2. Facial exercises. 3. Face—Care and hygiene. 4. Facial expression. I. Title.
[RA778.E396   1999]
646.7'26—dc21   98-50593
                                                                              CIP

First St. Martin's Griffin Edition: July 1999
10 9 8 7 6 5 4 3 2 1

This book is dedicated to

my beloved daughter

Karin

and to our memory of

Kirsten.

Contents

Contents
_____

viii

Acknowledgments

Professional

Janet Nager—whose belief in me and our work allowed this book to come into fruition

Reagan Arthur—my editor, for excellence

Cynthia Merman—my copy editor, for very helpful editing

Wendy Keller—my agent, who put it all together . . . so quickly!

Ariela Briagh Wilcox—for orchestrating the book proposal

Joel Isaacs, Lisbeth Marcher, and *BodyNamics*—for truth and wisdom about the life of our bodies

Donna Eden—my friend, for acupressure wisdom

Barbara Roberts—for Chinese face reading instruction

Robert Frost and Marilyn Davies—for photography

Helen Redman—for illustrations

Susan Cox of Cox Productions—for computer graphics

Karin Brock—for help in the very beginning

All my clients—the most valuable of resources

Personal

Bob and Marina—for redefining friendship

Acknowledgments

x

Anellina—for such patient nurturing

Damon and Chelsea—for drawing me from my complacency back into life

Gregg Tiffen—for showing the way to a life that makes sense

Dorothea—for inspiring me to mature, not get old

Britt—for Montana

Introduction

Years ago, when youth gave me my toned body and face effort-
lessly, I was struck by the natural beauty of my friend Dorothea,
then in her seventies. "How do you do it?" I asked in a moment
of candor. She paused and said with Katharine Hepburn forth-
rightness, "When I see someone whose aging I admire, I say,
'That's me!' and when I see the opposite, I say, 'Not me!'" I have
always remembered her words and followed them.

Timeless Face, a minutes-a-day facial toning program, is one
outcome of this decision. As a book, it is divided into two parts.
Part I gives an overview of Chinese face reading and explains acupressure, with two illustrations. Part II is the Timeless Face program, with chapters on each area of the face and twenty-three
facial toning exercises illustrated with photos.

Timeless Face will show you how to have a more beautiful,
toned, and open face in just minutes a day. I've combined the
most effective facial toning exercises with the wisdom of Chinese
face reading and the use of acupressure points to activate energy
and circulation in the face. Each exercise outlines the practical
tools required to move lethargy to action, stress to relaxation, fa-

tigue to excitement, wariness to receptivity—to name a few—while a beautifully toned face emerges. Through this innovative program, you will develop a more youthful and open face. As you tone using the easy-to-understand steps of my program, you will have the opportunity to learn from ancient wisdom how your face affects the alliance of body, mind, and spirit.

What is Chinese face reading? And why will it provide such a powerful dimension to facial toning? Over the centuries, Chinese traders put together, through careful observation, a uniquely insightful way of understanding the people with whom they were trading. They "read" their faces, interpreting expressions, the subtle movement of muscles, and each face's unique structure. This technique enabled a person to read others like an open book. This, of course, enhanced the worldwide reputation of the Chinese as shrewd and clever traders.

Chinese face reading offers us not only an effective tool with which to understand others more fully but also a very powerful tool for self-development. For example, the Chinese believe face reading teaches that the area of the eyes expresses the soul and governs the ability to be clear-sighted in complex situations. An exercised eye area increases your ability to improve your skill in these areas, while it also tones away puffiness, droops, and lackluster eyes.

The nose is seen as the energy source of the body. Exercising my nose has never failed to increase my physical energy—even when my reservoirs seemed dried up.

As with all ancient wisdom, the more you explore it, the deeper it gets. Your toning will relieve the signs of stress and time in your face and increase your awareness of yourself in the presence of your life.

Your face greets the world. Through the face, you give a strong impression of yourself and receive the same impressions from others. When face-to-face with ourselves, we are often surprised by what we see. Sometimes through a candid photo, an unexpected mirror, or another's comments, we may realize that our face does not accurately convey our inner experience of ourself. And we end up exclaiming, "That's not me, is it?"

I followed my friend Dorothea's advice, spurred on by photos, and I kept my program to myself. Not from a need to hoard the knowledge, but more from embarrassment that the exercises required "funny" faces. I was raised in a home where the maintenance of the face and body was seen as less important than other pursuits. So quietly, with the bathroom door closed, I contorted my face. Happy with the results, but not sure of the value of sharing them, I lived my life.

What woman or man doesn't want to look and feel "right"—to know that the outer self truly reflects the inner self? All of us have an inner picture of ourselves we cherish, one that is built on the reality of our bone structure and age, a picture that holds our own inner ideal. Many of us fall prey to an external idea of what we should look like. Confronted by so many idealized, enhanced images of physical beauty in film, television, and advertising, we can lose our "inner" picture. But that picture is there, and it is your deep inner wisdom saying, "If I used *all* my natural potential, this is how I would look."

In the 1970s, I saw a film in which one woman said to another, "Do you ever feel as if you were raised never to be over forty?" The truth of this hit me like a ton of bricks. At that moment, I made up my mind that my life would go beyond forty and that I would embrace the years ahead and welcome their potential for grace, dignity, beauty, and fun.

Just as one approaches any great journey with guidelines, priorities, and goals, maturing must also be approached with vision. Certainly, maturing is one of life's most intimate experiences— and a privilege not granted to all. As with any intimate experience, it encompasses a myriad of facets: personal development, family commitments, friendship choices, business contributions, and our spiritual path. Each one of these, theoretically, improves our own personal quality. Our quality, integrated, allows us to glow like a candle in a dark room.

Timeless Face acknowledges the effects of emotion on your face. How often have you seen someone and been stunned by how much he has aged? Or seen someone who has been through great stress and noticed the emotion frozen on her worn face? A healthy, fluid face will always show love, fear, joy, pain, excitement, depression, fatigue. For those of us on the facial toning program, these emotions flow easily *through* our faces, without imprisoning our countenance in a set expression.

Remember that warm smile from a loved one that set your heart aglow? Warmth, happiness, the reward of a full, rich facial expression filled with life and emotion—this wonderful smile is seen most often on a child's face because it is free of any but the current emotion. There are no holdovers from yesterday's pain or last year's disappointment.

We don't want unpleasantly set faces. We buy makeup and change our hairstyle to enhance our face. What we fail to realize or acknowledge is that it is an open, fresh face we long for, but we don't know how to keep it or get it back. Life goes on and on—through feast and famine—and each experience becomes a part of you. But once you start the Timeless Face program you will be filled with a renewed belief that time and stress can *help* you. They are part of life's banquet, and you can look great *because* of—not in spite of—them.

As you seek the face of others and your face is sought by them, you will never have to be unsure again.

I have a client who cared for her ill husband for the last five years of his life. After he died, she was shocked when she looked in the mirror and saw a worn old woman.

She began my Timeless Face program, and within only ten days her sad and tired face was regaining liveliness. As she continued the program, she was rewarded by a return to her countenance of humor, so much a part of her nature, and her eyes began to dance again. Her face became toned and her spirit shone through. She maintains her exercises to this day. Her confidence in herself continues to increase as she creates a life in which she flourishes.

Take a minute with yourself and a hand mirror. Allow your face to settle into repose. Relax your facial muscles into the face you drive with, listen with, read a book with—the face you wear 80 percent of the day. Is this what you want? Is this you? Or would you like to be something else? Happier, more alive, curious, fresh, more open, more *yourself.* Not just one narrow part of you.

When I work with my clients, I ask them to look honestly at the "greeting" of their faces. Is their face in repose true to their inner picture, the self they want to wear when they say hello to the world? Or is that face a limited, closed expression of themselves? Each client I have worked with has come in with her own very personal story and goal.

Janet was one of my first clients, a woman in her midforties with a remarkable face that combines strength and beauty. She came to me because her upper lip was barely visible. We immediately started on the Timeless Face program, focusing on the exercise that would release the muscles and balance the tone of the upper lip. Just one week later, Janet came to her session with a fuller upper lip. The mouth's influence on the ability to nurture also allowed Janet a more nurturing expression and feeling toward herself and others.

Stephanie is a lovely woman in her midthirties whose face conveys the nobility of her Aztec ancestors. However, she also inherited a very strong tendency for the cheeks and the corners of the mouth to droop. She launched enthusiastically into the program to tone her cheeks and bring the corners of her mouth into a more pleasing upward swing. Her progress in six weeks showed a very noticeable improvement: The cheeks are now far more defined, and the mouth in repose wears a pleasant expression. As her mouth has lifted, laughter has become more a part of her life.

Kathy is a woman in her late twenties who had a troubled childhood. Kathy was unhappy that her face, when relaxed, always looked sad. We planned a balanced overall program with an emphasis on the eyes and cheeks. In just a few weeks, Kathy saw her countenance lift and open, and as her face changed, her level of confidence increased. Kathy remains a daily faithful practitioner of the Timeless Face program.

Marla is a woman in her fifties who had a successful career in the military. However, the years of discipline had etched a severity in her face. She longed for a softer, more receptive appearance. Marla practiced the complete program and found that, in a few months, her face had lost its set look and now looked "fresher" and more youthful.

The face, emotionally loaded or free and open, is contoured by bone and muscles underlying the skin. As certain emotions register and are expressed often, some muscles become chronically underused and others chronically overused. The outcome of this slow imbalance and decline of definition is what we call "natural aging."

There is nothing natural about it. What we call natural aging is poor muscle tone and poor muscle balance in the underpinning of the skin.

A regularly exercised face, like a regularly exercised body, stays contoured and defined; *this* is *natural* aging—the face you are meant to have. I have avoided cosmetic surgery, and I find face exercise is the commonsense middle ground between the unexercised face and facial surgery. Facial surgery is not a panacea, as the face can looked skinned without underlying muscle tone.

My most challenging year was 1995. I call this "front-line"

work, applying all my self-knowledge and self-maintenance effectively to shape a life in which I, and those I love, flourish. My precious oldest daughter, Kirsten, died suddenly, and I am now a grandma-mama, helping to raise my two grandchildren, Chelsea, six, and Damon, eleven.

For the first few months, my well-ordered life, my face, and my body were a wreck. Step by step, my family and I are shaping a new life. Without my program and my beliefs, I would now still be worn, sad, and stressed with no way to turn it around. Timeless Face has given me a greater understanding of the wellspring of resources available in ancient wisdom when joined with Western applications. My optimism has returned, my face has lost its mask of grief, and I am becoming once again open and enthusiastic.

I have learned that the body, mind, and spirit absolutely do reflect each other, the face included!

The Timeless Face program is an exciting adventure into the world of facial toning. Instead of fearing time for its effects on your face, the life events that occur over time become the agents to improve your facial tone and countenance. You face your life with confidence and presence. For the first time, you will learn how your feelings affect your face, and you will learn what to do about it so your facial toning exercises will then affect positively how you feel—about yourself and about your life!

On this facial toning program there are no boring, repetitious exercises. They've been banished forever, replaced by facial movements that have meaning and relevance.

I have devoted myself to helping people enjoy their lives more as they live and love. This program is the product of years of experimentation, observation, and study. I first applied the combination of facial toning, body-based therapy, and Eastern wisdom to myself, then to my friends, and finally to clients, refining it constantly. The result is a facial toning program so logical and so simple that you will wonder why it wasn't thought of before. The Timeless Face program isn't a magic ticket to youth. It is not a temporary plan that creates a permanent change. It is a facial toning program for each individual. This is a program you make your own.

There is a potential loveliness and vitality inherent in all humanity, and we have a wonderful opportunity, even joyous responsibility, to embrace our own uniqueness as we grow and learn to flourish through life and its events. Our natural birthright is a toned and open face, ready for the great journey!

And now let's unveil your Timeless Face.

PART I

Overview

Chapter 1

Chinese Face Reading

*I*magine, for a moment, that you live in a country governed absolutely by rules, traditions, and status. You have been taught from infancy a discipline of body and face that creates controlled composure at all times. Your hands are hidden in your sleeves. Your conversation is polite. Your clothes and status alone speak for you, and you forgo all individuality for this rigid structure.

In this enigmatic culture you also need to live a life. To do this, you need to understand whom you can trust and whom you cannot trust, how to have love relationships based on honesty, and how to be successful in the world by understanding the needs and natures of others.

This was the dilemma of old China. After centuries of rigid rules and traditions, this culture idolized a form and discipline that closed one's individual spontaneous nature to self-expression— yet understanding others was as pertinent then as it is today. Within the challenges of these circumstances, understanding the nature of others became an artful skill of interpreting a person's only visible clues—the face. Chinese traders became particularly skilled at this craft. Face reading was a grassroots skill, born from observation, driven by the need to succeed, passed from generation to generation, information as valuable as gold.

We all know that even the most controlled face can show deeply felt emotions or reactions: the pupil of an eye contracting with fear, dilating with pleasure; a mouth tightening with displeasure, relaxing with trust; a chin held back with suppressed tears, thrust forward in aggression. Over the centuries in China, reading these facial reflexes was expanded to include the *meaning* in a face's structure, feature placement, and contour.

Chinese face reading works. Centuries of observation have been honed into a marvelous tool to better understand one another.

I have turned the tables a bit. I have taken the wisdom of those long-ago traders, coupled it with Western facial toning techniques and body-based therapy, and created Timeless Face, a blending of East and West. This program is a quantum leap forward that takes the observation of *others* and applies it directly to the development of the *self.*

By following the wisdom of face reading I learned, for instance, that deep furrows from the nose to mouth represent suppressed emotions and express a tendency to take ones responsibilities *very* seriously. I wondered, if I exercised the muscles under this area, would I then notice a difference in my ability to speak up for myself, and would I lighten my responsibilities by bringing more of my needs and nature into them? My answer was certain. As the lines smoothed out, so did I. I became more relaxed within my life's responsibilities and more able to express myself, instead of viewing my responsibilities as more important than me. A balance was occurring.

I then started to apply more ideas. Would getting rid of the bags under my eyes make me more lighthearted? Would exercising my mouth enable me to speak more caringly without self-compromise? Suddenly I entered a whole new world of toning through understanding the face's effect on the body, mind, and spirit.

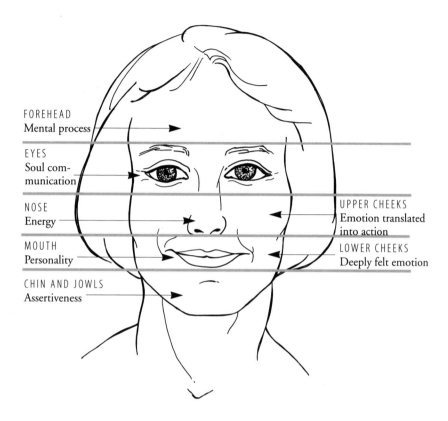

FOREHEAD
Mental process

EYES
Soul com-
munication

NOSE
Energy

MOUTH
Personality

CHIN AND JOWLS
Assertiveness

UPPER CHEEKS
Emotion translated
into action

LOWER CHEEKS
Deeply felt emotion

Using experiences gained through my lifelong fascination with energy, health, and the body, I began to include some acupressure points in my toning regime. I developed a program blending the best of the East and West and was pleased with the result! My face was aging with a natural, balanced look.

If another's drooping mouth means dissatisfaction, then the same is true for you and me. In my program you exercise and tone the involved muscles and deepen the toning by holding energy points. As the muscles around the mouth regain their natural balance with one another, this unhappy downward turn uplifts to a pleasant openness, and you feel more optimistic in your life as a direct result.

You are out to dinner with a loved one and want to encourage openness. Using the principles of Timeless Face, you relax the toned muscles around the eyes and lift the lid slightly. Voilà, the evening opens like a flower. Or you want to create the opposite ambiance—more protective—so you do the reverse with your eyes, all very subtly, and you are more contained, more controlled.

It becomes second nature simply to call on this most natural animated communicator of yourself, your face. You tone, relax, allow your natural inner countenance to emerge, and your view of life alters. Life hasn't changed—*you* have, and so life changes favorably in its response to you.

Chapter 2

Why Acupressure?

$\mathcal{A}$cupressure is a self-balancing technique that comes from China. It has been used for thousands of years as a tool for improving health, emotional balance, and physical vitality. Through pressure or massage at certain points on the skin, acupressure stimulates energy that flows within the body. These points are identified by number in the acupressure points chart (pages 8–9). As you stimulate these points as a part of your exercise routine, you will engage the energetic flows to improve energy, skin tone, emotional balance, and openness on the face. As a result, the job of restoring open, toned balance to your face gets done better, with longer-lasting results.

I have chosen these particular acupressure points because of their unusual effectiveness and their power to balance the inner emotional life as it reflects on your face.

I found that in doing the Eye Crunch exercise, my undereye puffiness decreased and so did some of my heavyheartedness. Then, by doing the Eye Crunch while stimulating acupressure points 1 and 3, I developed more sparkle in my eyes and im-

ACUPRESSURE POINTS

The stimulation of these points brings in vitality to improve skin tone and replaces the emotionally set face with an open countenance of well-being.

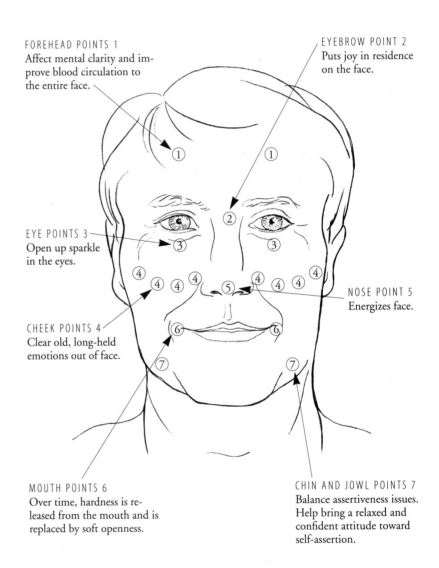

FOREHEAD POINTS 1
Affect mental clarity and improve blood circulation to the entire face.

EYEBROW POINT 2
Puts joy in residence on the face.

EYE POINTS 3
Open up sparkle in the eyes.

NOSE POINT 5
Energizes face.

CHEEK POINTS 4
Clear old, long-held emotions out of face.

MOUTH POINTS 6
Over time, hardness is released from the mouth and is replaced by soft openness.

CHIN AND JOWL POINTS 7
Balance assertiveness issues. Help bring a relaxed and confident attitude toward self-assertion.

Forehead Points 1

For mental clarity	Hold points 1 with the tips of your first and second fingers lightly for up to one minute, or until you feel the rhythm of a light pulse under your fingertips balance on both sides into an even pulse.
For improved circulation throughout the entire face	Stretch your forehead skin vertically, then horizontally, three to five times. First, place your fingertips on the right and left sides of the forehead at the hairline, gently stretch the skin. Second, place your fingertips on your upper hairline and eyebrows and gently stretch the skin. This takes about five seconds.

Eye and Eyebrow Points 2 and 3

To put delight and joy in residence on the face	Start at point 2 with the tips of the first and second fingers of each hand applying upward pressure and slowly fan out over your forehead. This is good anytime but is most effective when you are feeling joyful, delighted, and magical. Do this two to ten seconds.
To bring sparkle into your eyes by increasing your comfort in your life	Press points 3 gently with your fingertips, as before, for up to one minute.

Cheek and Nose Points 4 and 5

Letting go clears emotions and creates a soft, pleasant face when used over time	Press firmly with the fingertip of your index finger along points 4, massaging first to your right, then to your left. Do this for ten to thirty seconds.
Increases physical energy sand facial vitality	Take hold of your nose tip at point 5 and masage. Pressing on the tip, rotate counterclockwise and then clockwise, up to one minute.

Mouth Points 6

Soften the mouth by releasing inner and outer judgments held in the tissue	Purse the corners of your mouth against your teeth. Press points 6 firmly with the tips of your index finger, massaging first to your right, then to your left, for ten to fifteen seconds. NOT FOR PREGNANT WOMEN.

Chin and Jowl Points 7

Balances assertiveness with a relaxed, confident attitude	Hold points 7 softly and release the jaw back down. Slack-jawed, hold for thirty seconds to one minute.

proved my mental clarity. Over time these effects became more and more apparent.

The acupressure points can also be used independently. For example, point 2, between the eyebrows, will serve you best when stimulated by pressing between the eyebrows and then stretching the skin in an upward fanning motion while you are experiencing joy, elation, and delight. Although it is a bit weird to massage between your eyebrows at this time, this point infuses the face with these pleasurable expressions, allowing them to rest on your face for more than a fleeting magic moment. The more you do it, the more your face shines with delight.

Each point in the chart is powerful in its ability to increase the desired energy flow. There is, however, one important exception. When a woman is pregnant, it is not advisable to release a downward flush of energy. Points 6 at the corners of the mouth help to drain and flush away old feelings. Since it is a downward movement, don't do it if you are pregnant.

PART II

Timeless Face Program

C h a p t e r   3

Before You Begin:
An Exercise Preview

P o i n t s   t o   R e m e m b e r

1. Lightweight surgical tape placed over or alongside areas to be exercised will help smooth your skin while you exercise the underlying muscles. Strategically placing fingers around or on the area to be exercised is an option you might choose to help slow down skin lining in certain areas of concern to you.

2. You breathe oxygen and circulation into the skin. Breathe, breathe, breathe.

3. If your skin feels dry, a little of your favorite cream applied before exercising is a good idea.

4. These are small muscles. They don't need to be worked a lot, and they are all very interconnected. Work one group and your whole face will feel it. Beginner or advanced, do the same number of repetitions. The goal is to return natural balance and tone to the muscles of your face. This is accomplished through gentle muscle movement and acupressure

stimulation, which combine to develop your awareness of your facial muscles. It is this awareness that separates the beginner from the advanced—not the ability to do repetitions.

5. I believe the reason facial exercise hasn't caught on—even though it certainly works—is that the face holds so much emotion and tension that as you exercise certain muscle groups, the emotion releases and you may feel uneasy. Unprepared for this, the tendency is to avoid the cause. Not enough time, can't understand it, and doesn't work fast enough are some of the frequent rationales for stopping. Expect to have some uneasy feelings, pangs, old memories, stiffness, and other reactions. They pass quickly and are a natural part of your own fresh face emerging from under its frozen layer. Soon your face will feel flexible, not stiff, and will be filled with your own animation.

6. You may find that the muscles under the areas where your skin has lines respond and tone better when given a light stretching before exercising. Gently pull on the muscle lengthwise and then widthwise as best you can. Just be gentle! The muscles under puffiness gain elasticity better when simply exercised. The stretching returns length and elasticity to overly tight muscles—held in chronic tension—thus contributing to lining. And the exercising returns tone and elasticity to muscles with low elasticity. The low elasticity contributes to the poor tone of puffing and bags.

7. All of these exercises are more effective, albeit more difficult, if you lie down with your head lifted up, unsupported, one or two inches.

8. One real problem with face exercises is jaw tension. Most of us tense the jaw for everything and hold the jaw in chronic tension. Learn the correct position of your jaw, which can be maintained for all but a few mouth and jaw exercises. The positioning is as follows: Allow your jaw to relax back, as if you were deeply asleep or "looking dumb." Lips are separated.

This is the correct position for a relaxed jaw: back and then naturally dropping down. Now position the tip of your tongue on your palate behind your two front teeth. As you do the exercises, your jaw will move but be in a better position for the movement and be less inclined to grit. Again, almost all the exercises can be done with this positioning. The tip of your tongue holds the jaw in place, enabling you to exercise your face without loading your jaw with tension.

9. You will have what I call "body echoes" when you do your face program. These echoes vary for each person. Some find their little fingers curled when they exercise their eyes. Some may feel their shoulders tighten when they do the jaw exercises. Many feel warmth and aliveness throughout the body while exercising the mouth. These are examples of the face being a part of the body-mind-spirit alliance. Some echoes will lessen as you progress, as you will have, in some cases, freed your body from tension habit patterns that are counterproductive to an active, high-energy life.

10. Stimulate acupressure points before exercising to energize the muscles, or afterward to drain out the old, accumulated energy.

11. The human characteristics identified with the muscle groups do not imply that every person necessarily has every characteristic listed. For instance, someone with bags may be holding in grief but might not be at all weakened in her ability to concentrate and consider. Find your own unique patterns, with this book as a guide.

12. There are many physical reasons for stress and time to show on our faces. These are well known: food, drink, drugs, cigarettes, genetics, sun, weight issues, medications to name a few. I don't address these factors in this book, not because they are not important, but because this book is about life's experience and its effect on us, how that is reflected in our faces, and what to do about it.

13. You will very often find one side of your face is easier to exercise than the other. This is normal and will even out as you progress.

Every exercise in the Timeless Face program contains the following information:

Benefits: How this exercise will affect your face physically.

Expression: The facial expression that, when mimicked, will help you to isolate the muscle to be exercised. To use the natural expressive qualities of your face, think of a real event in your life and let your face express it. The expression will activate, with less effort, the muscle you are preparing to isolate and exercise.

Muscle: The name of the muscle or muscles you are exercising

Time: A realistic number of repetitions needed to get results. As you become more advanced, you don't increase repetitions. But you become more adept at subtle facial toning, conscious of the effect of your face on your world.

Causes: How your life's events and your attitudes—mental, emotional, and spiritual—affect your face.

Corrects: The mental, emotional, and spiritual areas that will be enhanced and balanced through the program.

Wise application: An idea for integrating the program into your daily life.

The exercise: What to do and how to do it.

Associated acupressure points: Instructions for the best way to activate them.

Illustrations: How you will look while doing the exercise.

Chapter 4

Forehead

*T*he forehead shows our particular orientation to intelligence. A high forehead indicates a strong, thinking mind. A low forehead indicates a reliance on instinctive intelligence. Acupressure points 1 help create greater mental clarity.

FOREHEAD LIFT

Benefits: Stops the drooping of the forehead, which squashes the eyebrows and reduces the size of your eyes. Smooths the forehead and restores arch and shape to eyebrows.

Expression: "Let me think. I'll get the answer to this question."

Muscle: Frontalis

Time: Seven to ten repetitions

Causes: The lines on the forehead and drooping eyebrows are caused by:

- overfocusing
- worry
- anxiety
- fear
- lack of (or overseeking for) mental clarity

Corrects: This exercise will:

- improve mental clarity
- improve confidence in your intelligence
- bring mental calm, especially when you simultaneously hold acupressure points 1 lightly for one minute
- bring greater vision in decision making and belief in the future

Wise application: When you are having a problem with repetitive and stale thinking, lightly hold acupressure points 1 for one minute or more. Your mind will be clearer and more refreshed.

"Let me think. I'll get the answer to this question." Notice the eyebrows are lifted up and wide.

1. Position your jaw and tongue.

2. Place your index fingertips just above your eyebrows and gently press down.

3. Slowly lift and push your eyebrows *high* and *wide*. High is easier than wide, but both are necessary to get the full benefits of the exercise. Slowly relax your eyebrows back to their natural position. Lifting your eyebrows wide is a subtle movement and thinking them wide helps activate the appropriate muscle.

4. Repeat seven to ten times.

Acupressure points 1: Rest your fingertips lightly for one minute, or until you feel a light pulse.

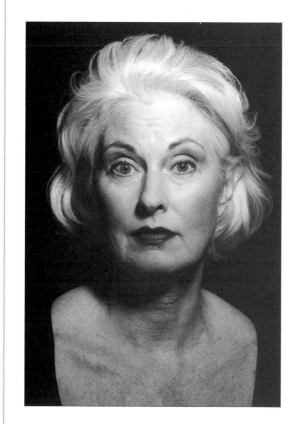

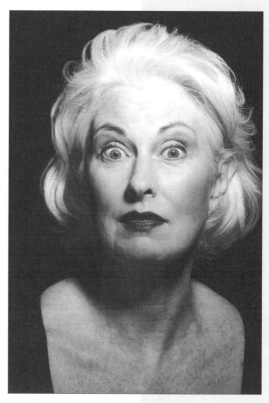

Eyes

*T*he eyes are the communicator of the soul. Large eyes show an openness and receptivity to life; small eyes donate a cautious and contained approach to life. Exercising the muscles of the eye segment provides balance between openness and containment. The acupressure points 3, when properly stimulated will, over time, fill the eyes with the sparkle of your aliveness and presence.

DESQUINTER

Benefit:	Smooths the vertical lines between the eyebrows.
Expression:	Perplexed: "What do you mean, 20 percent interest?"
Muscle:	Corrugator supercilii
Time:	Seven to ten repetitions
Causes:	Squint lines between the eyes are the result of:

- confusion
- concern
- concentration
- controlling issues

Corrects:	This exercise will:

- bring clarity into confusion
- move concentration into creative application
- help you recognize opportunity as it appears
- increase your ability to have vision

Wise application:	If you need to be aware of your options and make a clear, focused decision, do repetitions of the Desquinter.

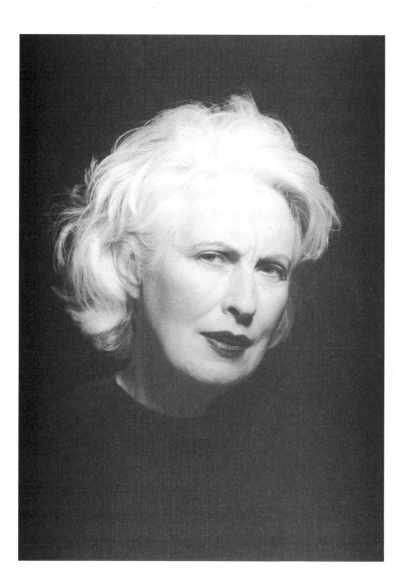

Perplexed. The eyebrows are drawn into midline between the eyebrows above the nose.

1. Position your jaw and tongue.

2. Place two fingertips between your eyebrows and gently press apart from one another.

3. Bring your attention to a spot right between your eyebrows, eyes open. Squint, frown, and feel your muscles contract into that spot. Now use the muscles under your eyebrows to smooth out the vertical lines, lifting up high and wide out. Wide is a subtle movement—just thinking about it will activate the appropriate muscle.

4. Repeat seven to ten times.

Acupressure point 2: Rest your fingertips lightly on point 2 and then fan up high and out wide onto your forehead.

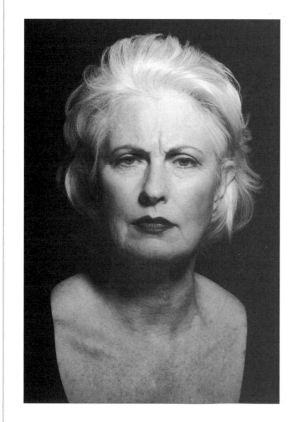

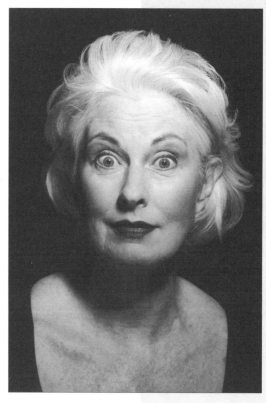

EYE CRUNCH

Benefit:	Tones the areas surrounding the eyes.
Expression:	Eyes tightly shut: "I'm not peeking!"
Muscle:	Orbicularis oculi
Time:	Seven to ten repetitions
Causes:	Loss of tone around the eyes is from:

- deeply felt sadness
- questions of what is real and what is not real
- flat, low energy eyes
- reduction in ability to appreciate a variety of visual impressions
- limiting your life options

Corrects: This exercise will:

- increase acceptance as you live with loss
- inspire confidence in yourself and your assessment of life
- increase spiritual intuition
- enable you to see that which is not obvious
- increase energy expression in your eyes
- enhance your ability to be visually influenced by life's beauty

Wise application: If you are feeling the changes of life very deeply and losing your sense of direction, the Eye Crunch will help open your inner vision and outer direction.

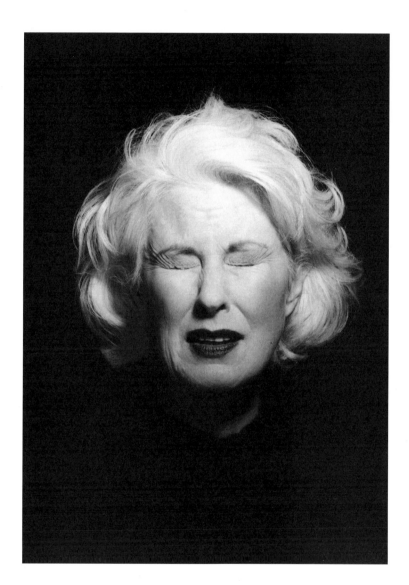

"I'm not peeking!" Eyes tightly squeezed shut.

1. Position your jaw and tongue.

2. Place two middle fingers between your eyebrows, pressing apart from one another slightly. Place your index fingers on the outside edge of your eyes as well.

3. Close your eyes. Slowly tighten the muscles around your eyes. Contracting these muscles more and more, letting the eyebrows lead, lift your upper lid and stretch way up. Slowly relax back into your eyes being simply closed.

4. Repeat seven to ten times:

Acupressure points 3: Light finger touch or tapping.

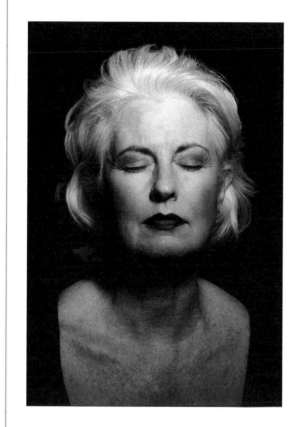

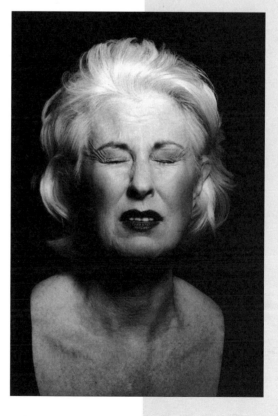

BAG REDUCER

Benefit:	Reduces under-eye puffiness.
Expression:	Unpleasant disbelief and puzzlement: "How can this be true?"
Muscle:	Orbicularis oculi, lower lid
Time:	Seven to ten repetitions
Causes:	Puffiness under the eyes is from:

- lack of deep and restful sleep
- grief not yet fully expressed
- desire to be buffered from life
- weakened ability to consider and contemplate

Corrects: This exercise will:

- improve your ability to see what is not obvious
- improve your ability to see your way through, one step at a time
- make your eyes more alive and expressive
- make life seem more positive and hopeful
- improve contemplation and consideration
- enhance spiritual intuition and vision

Wise application: When you are feeling discouraged, do the Bag Reducer twenty times. You will feel clearer about the best step to take next.

"How can this be true?" The lower eyelid is contracted—lifted up toward the eye.

1. Position your jaw and tongue.

2. Lightly touch your outer eye corners.

3. Close your eyes. Think about the expression and let your lower lid lift up. Keep the rest of your face relaxed. Hold for five counts. Relax back slowly.

4. Repeat seven to ten times.

Acupressure points 3: Light finger touch or tapping.

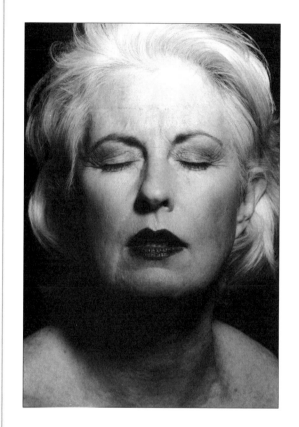

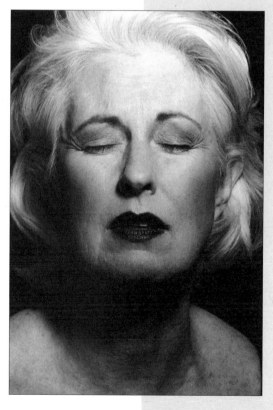

OPENER

Benefit:	Tones and firms the upper lid.
Expression:	Singing a great operatic aria with the eyes wide open, eyebrows up, blinking
Muscle:	Orbicularis oculi, upper lid
Time:	Seven to ten repetitions
Causes:	Loss of tone in the upper eyelid is from:

- emotional fatigue
- desire to withdraw from life
- life loss and deep sadness
- feeling like a martyr or a victim

Corrects:	This exercise will:

- bring a more bright, alert attitude
- create a deeper sense of presence and engagement
- open your receptivity and enthusiasm
- lift depression from early loss

Wise application:	If you don't like the situation you're in, and you want to protect your feelings, drop your upper lid down a bit.

Sing a great operatic aria. Just like a great diva singing a perfect high C, everything—mouth, eyes, and nose—is open wide and flared out. This expression tones the muscle at the top of the eyelid that holds the upper lid back where you want it.

1. Position your jaw and tongue.

2. Place your fingertips above your eyebrows, pressing down slightly.

3. Raise your eyebrows and close your eyes. Stretch upward with your eyebrows and stretch downward with your upper lids. Really stretch! You are creating maximum distance between your eyebrows and your eyelashes. Hold for a count of ten. Then very slowly relax.

4. Repeat seven to ten times.

Acupressure points 3: Light finger touch or tapping.

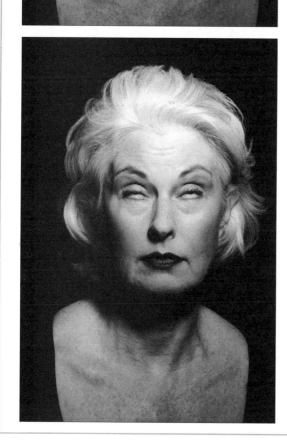

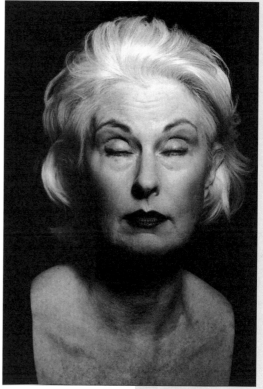

Benefit:	Lifts the upper lid for larger eyes.
Expression:	Surprise: confronted with something unexpected
Muscle:	Orbicularis oculi, upper lid
Time:	Seven to ten repetitions
Causes:	The eyelid loses tone from:

- boredom with life
- passive or closed mental attitude toward new information
- slowness to act on and trust your own instincts or intelligence
- procrastination

Corrects:	This exercise will:

- sharpen visual impressions
- improve your ability to be perceptive
- help you achieve balance in your timing and action
- enhance personal creativity
- appreciate timing as a tool for living

Wise application:	You have started to withdraw. Become more alert and present by doing the Upper Lid Toner. It is especially effective when combined with acupressure point 2.

Surprise. The eyebrows are high, as if they are lifting the upper lids up, while the lower lids pull down. As a result the eyes are fully open and may bulge a bit.

1. Position your jaw and tongue.

2. Place your fingertips above your eyebrows, pressing down gently.

3. Raise your eyebrows. Slowly, with as much control as possible, lower your upper lids and raise your lower lids. This looks like an eye squint without the scowl between your eyebrows. Your eyelids almost meet. Try to lower the upper lids and raise the lower at the same speed.

   Pull the upper lids up and back and at the same time think about making your eyes larger and larger. Try to raise and lower your lids at the same speed. It is as if you are trying to pull your whole ocular area back and away from something you're seeing but are unable to close your eyes to. Blink several times as you retain this stretch. Relax back slowly.

4. Repeat seven to ten times. This exercise requires more focus and awareness than the others. Keep at it. You can't be wrong and there is benefit in it all.

Acupressure point 2: Rest your fingertips lightly on point 2 and then fan up and out onto your forehead.

Acupressure points 3: Light finger touch or tapping.

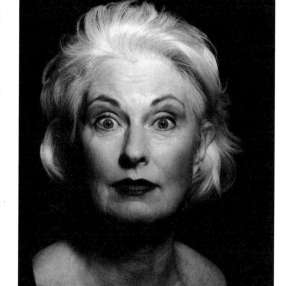

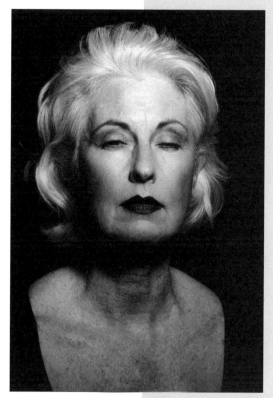

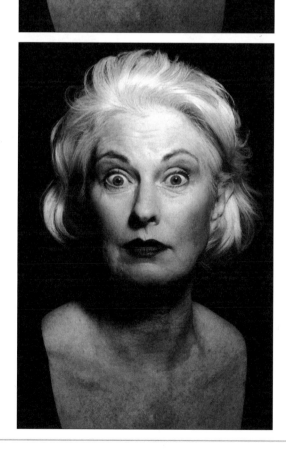

Benefit:	Alleviates puffy and drooping upper lids.
Expression:	"I need to rest and refocus."
Muscle:	Tensor tarsi
Time:	Seven to ten repetitions
Causes:	Puffy eyelids indicate:

- concern
- crying or needing to cry
- difficulty in mental concentration and retention
- a sense that life is overwhelming
- lack of energy in the eye

Corrects:	This exercise will:

- renew mental concentration and retention
- help you sort things out more easily
- improve energy and expression in the eye

Wise application:	You are tired and unfocused. Do The Thinker, gently squeezing and relaxing. Your eyes will refresh, and focus will return. This exercise works well with acupressure points 1.

"I need to rest and refocus." As you press gently on either side of the nose, you squeeze the inner and upper lids toward your fingers.

1. Position your jaw and tongue.

2. Place one finger between your eyebrows, pressing gently, then place your finger and thumb holding the sides of your nose at the tear ducts.

3. Close your eyes. Squeeze your eye muscles toward the bridge of your nose. Release the muscle slowly back to a normal position.

4. Repeat seven to ten times.

Acupressure points 3: Light finger touch or tapping.

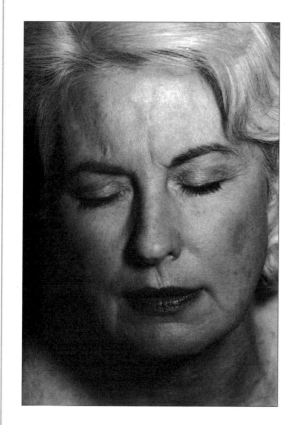

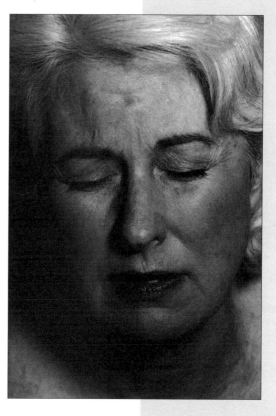

Chapter 6

Nose

The nose brings in breath, the life energy. Exercising the nose enhances and increases the energy available to your body. Your nose is like an engine; it just needs to be revved up occasionally.

Acupressure point 5 energizes the spine, bringing the face fresh vitality.

Benefits:	Smooths out the lines on the nose; fills in the valleys between the nose and cheek.
Expression:	Skepticism: you see something you doubt.
Muscles:	Procerus (nose); Levator quadratus labii superioris
Time:	Five to fifteen repetitions
Causes:	Problems with the nose result from:

- reduced or excessive sense of healthy competition in life
- feeling a loss of luster in life
- disgust
- apathy

Corrects: This exercise will:

- energize your body
- improve circulation and energetic flow to your face
- help you spiritually to see your place in life and how that is expressed in relationship to the things of this world
- energize and balance your activity level and assertion skills
- clarify your inner vision

Wise application: When you are feeling too low in your energy output, stimulate point 5 and exercise your nose to feel more energized.

Skepticism. Nostrils are flared out, eyebrows are lifted up, and a stretch is felt up the nose.

1. Position your jaw and tongue.

2. Place your fingertips pressing down above your eyebrows.

3. Flare your nostrils as big as you can and raise your eyebrows high and wide. Wrinkle your nose up—way up. Use your upper lip to pull your nose down as you keep your eyebrows high and wide. Even though they will come down, to some the effort to keep them high is an important part of the exercise.

4. Repeat five to fifteen times.

Acupressure point 5: Squeeze and massage the tip of your nose. Then, pressing on the tip, rotate to the right and then to the left.

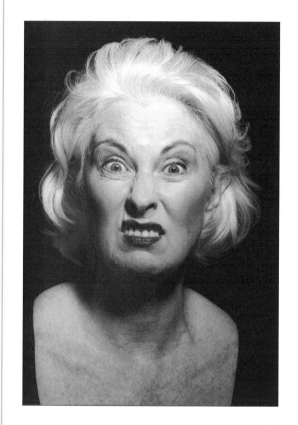

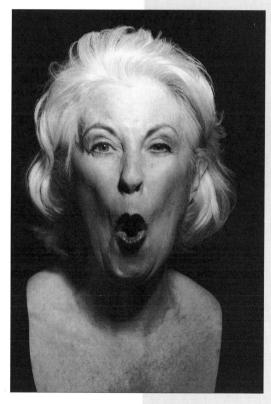

Chapter 7

Cheeks

The cheeks are divided into four areas: upper and lower, outer and inner. The upper cheek expresses personal action in the world. The lower cheek shows the personal inner relationship and deeply felt emotions. Gaunt cheeks indicate a separation from comfortable expression of deep emotions. Very full cheeks indicate a deeply felt emotional nature. The inner cheek plays a role in limiting perception. The outer cheeks are related to one's ability to expand one's life.

Acupressure points 4 lift long-held emotions off the face, creating, over time, a more pleasant countenance.

Benefit:	Firms and tones apple cheeks.
Expression:	Questioning interaction: "Do I want that?" Often humor is a part of the question.
Muscles:	Orbicularis oculi (lower section); the cheek muscles as a group
Time:	Five to fifteen repetitions
Causes:	The upper cheeks lose tone as a result of:

- lowering of self-reliance
- less risk taking
- self-doubt about choices and actions
- unclear understanding of where you fit harmoniously into life

Corrects:	This exercise will:

- move deep emotion into action
- increase self-reliance
- help you sort through extraneous information (with forehead lifted) to decide right action
- enhance an attitude of healthy quality control on your personal life

Wise application:	When you need a lift in your belief in yourself, do the Upper Cheek Lift in combination with acupressure points 4.

Questioning. The upper cheeks are lifted up, creating an apple cheek.

1. Position your jaw and tongue.

2. Lightly touch along your eyes.

3. Make an O with your mouth in such a way that no lines above your upper lip and from your nose to mouth are deepened. Squint your upper cheeks up as if you are trying to close your entire eyes with your cheeks by pressing them up. *Slowly* bring the cheek muscles down to their natural position.

4. Repeat five to fifteen times.

Acupressure points 4: Press firmly with your fingertips onto points 4, massaging in small circular motions to your right and then to your left.

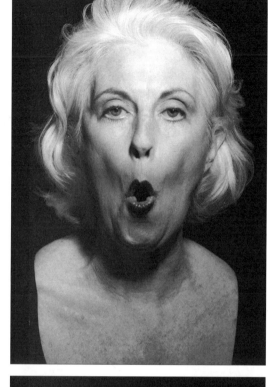

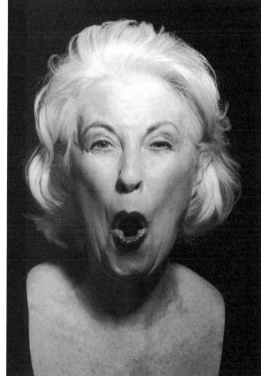

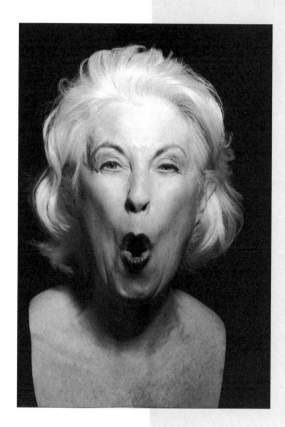

BALLOON

Benefit: Returns elasticity to the lower cheeks.

Expression: As kids you filled up your cheeks and then popped out the air.

Muscles: Zygomaticus major and minor

Time: Five to fifteen repetitions

Causes: The lower cheeks lose tone because:

- they are a holding tank for deeply held emotions
- passivity has become a way of life in order to escape from expressing deeply uncomfortable feelings
- if the cheek is gaunt, there is difficulty in knowing one's emotional nature, leading sometimes to insensitivity to self and others
- you are not living up to your creative potential

Corrects: Exercising the lower cheeks will:

- correct the inertia of deeply held emotions to allow for creative self-expression
- increase emotional receptivity
- allow natural emotions to have a fuller, richer impact, and create better emotional relationships

Wise application: When you begin to feel a bit "flat," the Balloon will give you a jump start.

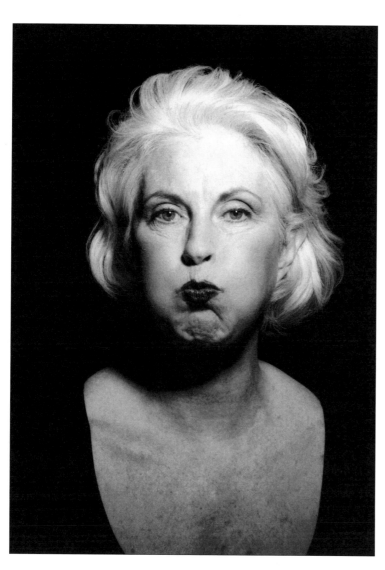

Fill your cheeks with air. Cheeks are filled up and rounded.

1. Position your jaw and tongue.

2. This is an isometric exercise using the breath and your cheek muscles in tension. Fill up one cheek to capacity with air. Now, using your cheek muscle, really push the air out. If you keep your lips tightly closed, the air provides resistance—muscles pushing in and finally winning as the air moves into your closed mouth. Fill up again and repeat until muscle feels fatigued. Repeat on the other side.

3. Repeat five to fifteen times.

Acupressure point 5: Squeeze and massage the tip of your nose. Next, pressing on the tip, rotate to the right and then to the left.

Acupressure points 6: Press firmly, massaging in small circular motion first to your right and then to your left.

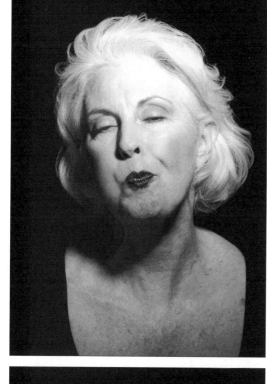

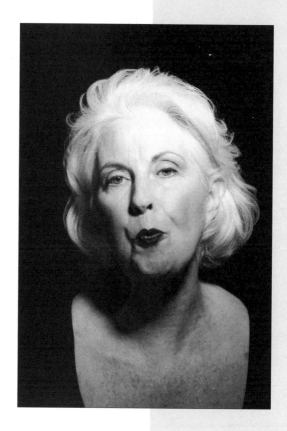

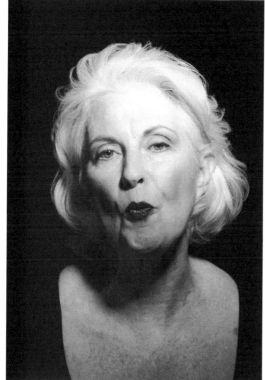

ERASING CARES

Benefit:	Decreases the nose-to-mouth furrow.
Expression:	Sweet smile with corners turning up
Muscles:	Lower orbicularis oris, caninus
Time:	Five to fifteen repetitions
Causes:	The nose-to-mouth furrow deepens as a result of:

- suppression of emotions
- feeling of being overburdened by responsibility
- feeling worn by life

Corrects: This exercise will:

- provide an attitude of lighthearted acceptance of pleasure in responsibilities
- assist communication and negotiation to express feelings of anger, fear, and guilt

Wise application: When you feel yourself become resigned, which means not seeing good alternatives, do Erasing Cares along with points 6. Relax your upper lip. You may be more able to enjoy the present or see how to alter it.

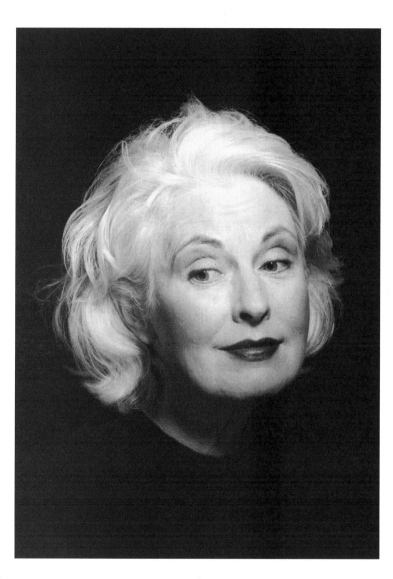

A sweet smile, corners turned up. Smile with outer corners of the mouth leading into the smile.

1. Position your jaw and tongue.

2. Make a tight grin, covering your teeth with your lips and pulling the corners of your mouth up. Keeping your teeth covered, make a pucker, really stretching out the muscles at the corners of your mouth. Return to the tight grin, again pulling the corners of your mouth up.

3. Repeat five to fifteen times.

Acupressure points 4: Press firmly with your fingertips onto points 4, massaging in small circular motions counterclockwise and then clockwise.

Acupressure points 6: Press firmly, massaging in small circular motions first to your right and then to your left.

Acupressure point 5: Squeeze and massage the tip of your nose and then, pressing on the tip, rotate to the right and then to the left.

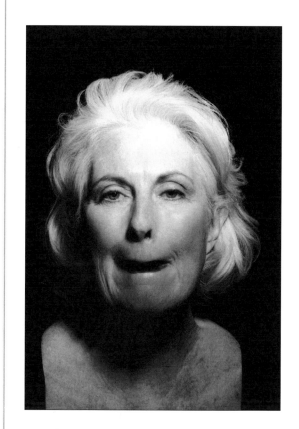

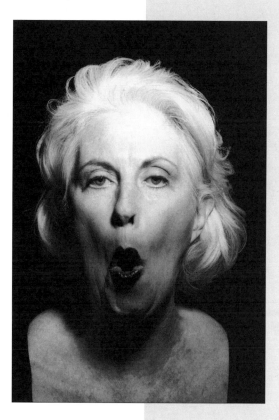

DETERMINED!

Benefit:	Firms and contours the sides of the face.
Expression:	Grit and determination
Muscle:	Masseter
Time:	Five to fifteen repetitions
Causes:	Jowls form on the face because of:

- suppressed emotion and anger
- a grin and bear it attitude
- a personality of great stubbornness

Corrects: This exercise will:

- divulge deeply held feelings
- allow more creative outlook in relating to the challenges of life
- help you let go of unnecessary control
- bring interest in communication and compromise
- reduce stress if used with points 7

Wise application: When you feel overly determined, clench your jaw once. Hold points 7 as you release your jaw down and back, letting it drop a little as if you are looking dumb.

Grit and determination. Jaw is gritted, mouth is firm, and nostrils are usually slightly flared.

1. Position your jaw and tongue.

2. Tense your underjaw by drawing your lower lip out into a grimace. Drop your head back slightly. Chew very slowly and deliberately *by letting your jaw relax back* and then slowly bringing your jaw up into a natural bite while holding the grimace. Relax and repeat.

   This exercise should be done with a *very* small range of motion, gradually increasing the range of your movement. This gentle approach can tone the masseter and reduce deeply held tension.

   This is a little tricky, but if you put your fingers on the masseter you will feel the muscles working. You may find your jaw more relaxed after you do this exercise slowly and easily.

3. Repeat five to fifteen times.

Acupressure points 6: Press firmly, massaging in a small circular motion first to your right and then to your left.

Acupressure points 7: Touch or tap lightly.

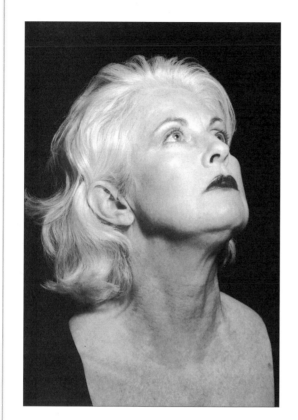

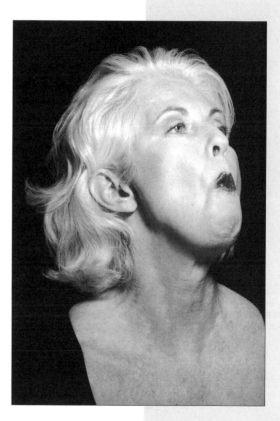

Mouth

The mouth tells of our personality. A soft, full mouth shows nurturing and supportive caring. A thin mouth denotes a practical and efficient person with very defined boundaries. Exercising the muscles in the mouth segment brings a balance between our nurturing characteristics and our practical boundaries. The acupressure points 4 release the energy from the heart center, arms, and hands. A connecting stream of warmhearted, practical, energetic potential fills your face, just waiting for you to hone and deliver it.

Benefits:	Lifts the outer and upper corners of the mouth. Helps to alleviate pouches at mouth corners.
Expression:	Prissy, self-righteousness
Muscle:	Risorius
Time:	Seven to ten repetitions
Causes:	Pouches or drooping at the corners of the mouth are caused by:

- self-esteem problems
- deep disappointments as yet unaccepted
- serious attitude toward responsibility that allows no self-nurturing
- ruminating
- power struggles: "I am a martyr" vs. "I am the authority"

Corrects:	This exercise will:

- increase self-acceptance
- encourage you to communicate more optimistically
- develop a lighter "spoonful of sugar" attitude toward life's challenges
- develop a deeper trust of your own decisions and ability to live with the outcome with greater confidence

Wise application:	Is your attitude toward something becoming tinged with disaster or displeasure? Do the Tight Grin to bring a lighter, more creative perspective, an uplift!

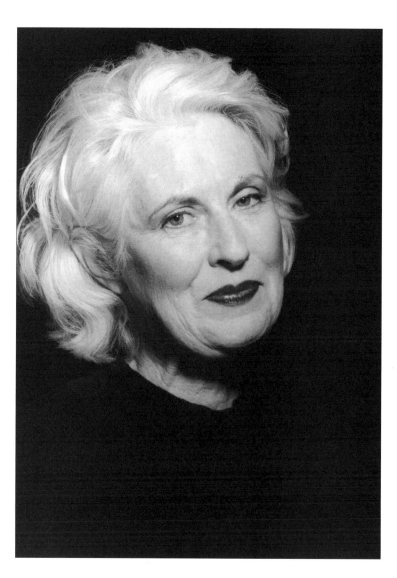

Prissy, self-righteous. The corners of the mouth are contracted against the teeth and turning up.

1. Position your jaw and tongue

2. Place the edges of your teeth together. Close your lips over your teeth, pressing the inner corners of your mouth against your teeth. This creates a tight, forced smile. Lift up the outer corners of your mouth. Keeping the tension against your teeth, make a big pucker. Now pull the corners of your mouth back up your teeth like a zipper. Maintain the tightness in the corners of your mouth throughout the exercise.

   It can be a little hard at the beginning to find these outer smile muscles. Bear with it and you will master it.

3. Repeat seven to ten times.

Acupressure points 6: Press firmly, massaging in small circular motions first to your right and then to your left.

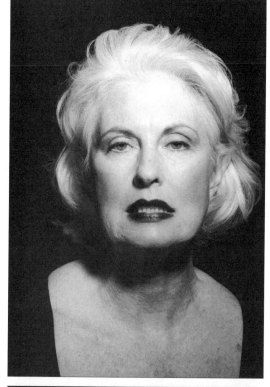

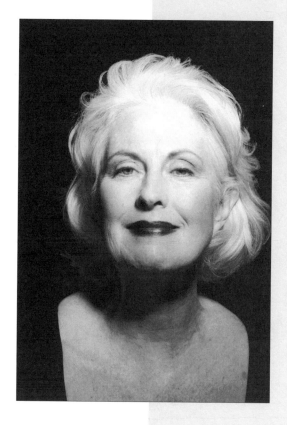

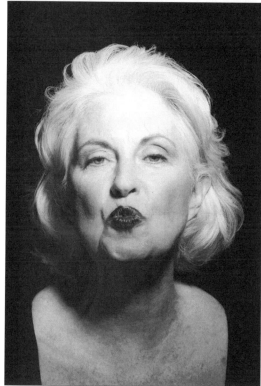

LIGHTHEARTED

Benefits:	Lifts the cheeks and corners of mouth; tones the upper lip.
Expression:	Joyous pleasure: "There is humor in all life!"
Muscles:	Zygomaticus major and minor
Time:	Five to fifteen repetitions
Causes:	Loss of tone in the outer corners of the mouth and lower cheeks is from:

- discouragement leading to loss of humor and laughter
- discontent with social life
- loss of confidence in life as a process of un-expected events
- fear-based smile

Corrects: This exercise will:

- lift your lower cheeks and mouth, creating a more pleasant countenance
- lift your mood as you find more pleasure within yourself, more spontaneous laughter
- make you happier with your social world
- help you feel more at home in your life
- reduce stress

Wise application: Life is looking somber, and you're taking your-self too seriously. Take a minute to exercise the zygomaticus—feel your viewpoint become more positive.

"There is humor in all life!" Have the entire upper lip lead into the smile—stretching the upper lip's smile by lifting the outer corners of the mouth.

1. Position your jaw and tongue.

2. The exercise is simple. Just put on a big smile and now make it bigger, eyes big, eyebrows high and wide. Emphasize the upper lip. Smile, lifting your mouth corners up and smile wide. Slowly relax.

3. Repeat five to fifteen times.

Acupressure points 6: Press firmly, massaging in small circular motions first to your right and then to your left.

Acupressure points 4: Press firmly with fingertips onto points 4, massaging in small circular motions to your right and then to your left.

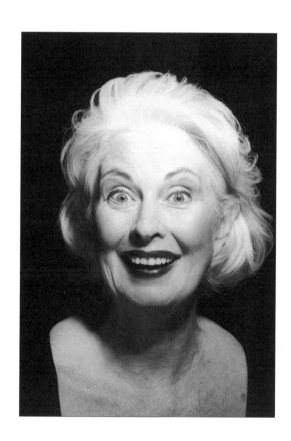

Benefits:	Firms and helps to smooth the upper lip. Helps to fill in mustache line, the horizontal line between the nose and upper lip that sometimes develops.
Expression:	Look at that!
Muscles:	Orbicularis oris and surrounding muscles
Time:	Five to fifteen repetitions
Causes:	The upper lip loses tone because of:

- silent disapproval
- weakening sexual energy
- shame in wanting physical pleasure
- disheartenment in relationships

Corrects:	This exercise will:

- enliven pelvic sensations
- energize your body's sensations of pleasure
- reach out in an invitation for contact

Wise application:	This a part of your face that has to do with physical pleasure. Exercising this muscle and energizing it will open pleasurable feelings and make you feel more alive.

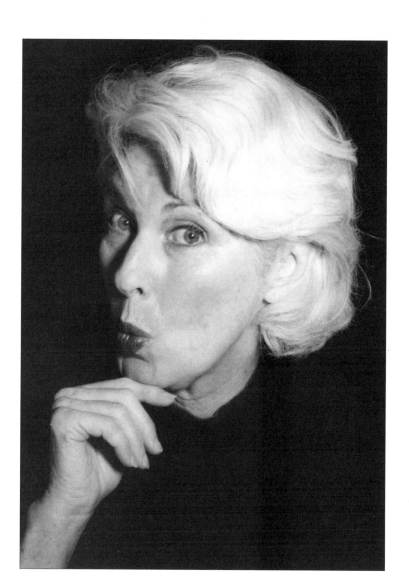

1. Position your jaw and tongue.

2. Imagine that you are pointing with the center of your upper lip. Tighten it more and more. You will feel your nostrils tighten a bit, too. Relax and repeat. This can be done in many repetitions if this is a problem area for you.

   In addition, if you have a mustache line, press down lightly in the center of the line as you do your exercise; the muscles there will work a little harder, thus helping to erase the line.

3. Repeat five to fifteen times.

Acupressure point 5: Squeeze and massage the tip of your nose and then, pressing on the tip, rotate to the right and then to the left.

Acupressure points 6: Press firmly, massaging in small circular motions first to your right and then to your left.

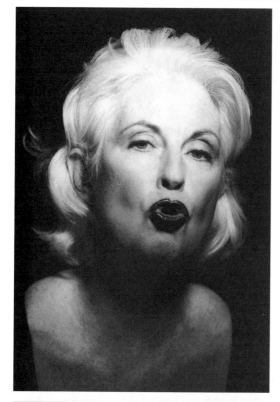

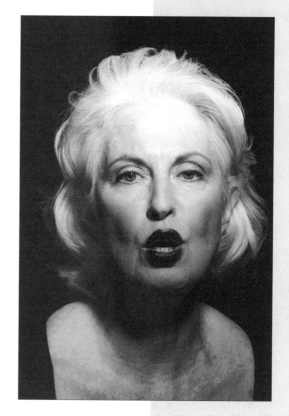

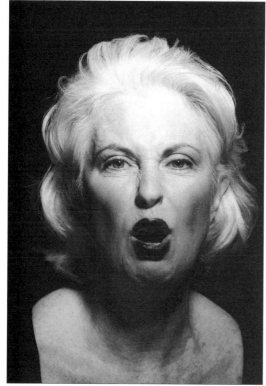

PUCKER, BLOW, AND BLOT

Benefits:	Tones the lips and increases circulation.
Expression:	Pucker: "Blow me a kiss!"
Muscle:	Orbicularis oris
Time:	Five to fifteen repetitions
Causes:	The lips lose fullness and tone when you:

- become more obsessed with efficiency and problem solving
- hide out in logical thinking rather than sharing emotionally
- don't express a full range of emotion vocally and verbally in an appropriate way
- lose vital interest in life
- lack trust in the love of others

Corrects: This exercise will:

- give you better ability to express your inner emotional life appropriately
- balance your sensuality with your efficient and focused life
- create warmth and strength in your smile
- reduce skepticism
- develop deeper ability for nurturing self and others

Wise application: If you want to have an open heart in a situation, allow your lips to become fuller. If you want to guard yourself, tighten your lips slightly under your teeth.

"Blow me a kiss!" Pucker up in a big fleshy pucker.

1. Position your jaw and tongue.

2. Give a big, juicy pucker and blow through it. Now blot your lips together, hiding your lips under your teeth while smiling.

3. Repeat five to fifteen times.

Acupressure points 6: Press firmly, massaging in small circular motions, first counterclockwise and then clockwise.

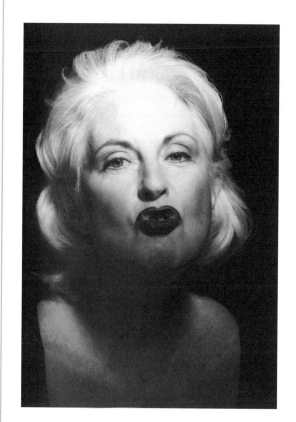

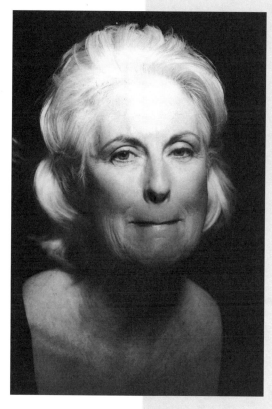

POOR BABY

Benefits:	Lessens the furrows from the mouth corners to the chin. Reduces lines on the chin.
Expression:	Humorous sympathy
Muscles:	Orbicularis oris, lower surrounding muscles
Time:	Five to fifteen repetitions
Causes:	Chin squiggles and lines from mouth to chin occur because of:

- suppression of childlike delight
- distaste
- displeasure
- pouting attitude
- withheld very old grief

Corrects:	This exercise will:

- smooth mouth-to-chin lines
- smooth out squiggle lines on the chin
- release some judgments and self-righteousness
- slowly move very old sad feelings

Wise application:	When you feel yourself becoming a little judgmental and displeased, lighten up your inner attitude with Poor Baby.

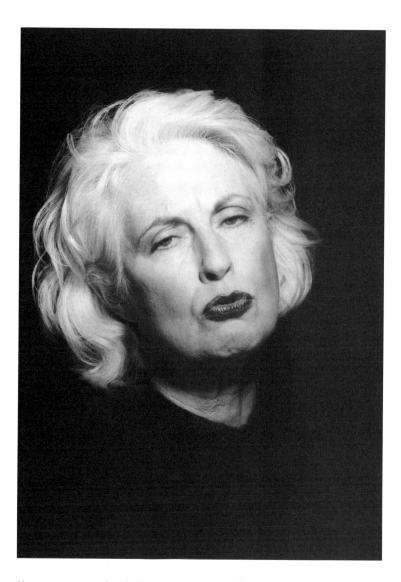

Humorous sympathy. The lower lip extends slightly and the corners of the
mouth turn down, as if you're saying, "Oh, you poor thing."

1. Position your jaw and tongue.

2. Turn down the corners of your mouth in a pout. Now draw them together as if trying to get the corners to meet in the middle. The lower lip will lift up and out. Relax out of it slowly.

3. Repeat five to fifteen times.

Acupressure points 7: Touch or tap lightly.

Acupressure points 6: Press firmly, massaging in small circular motion, first counterclockwise and then clockwise.

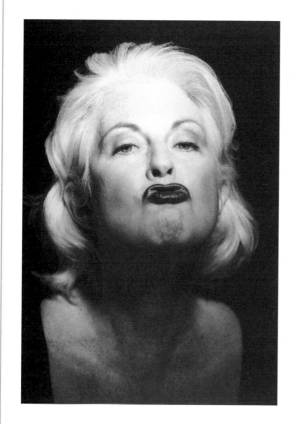

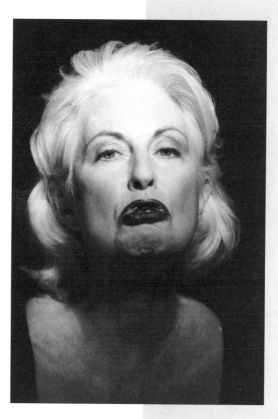

Jaw and Chin

The jaw and chin show the relationship to assertion. A jaw that is retracted tells of personal conflict about comfortably stepping forward to take one's place in life with confidence and ease. A jaw that is thrust forward generally shows aggressive and stubborn characteristics. Creating elasticity in the jaw area, and most particularly in the actual joint, restores balance and helps you know when to step forward on behalf of yourself and when to step back. Acupressure points 7 release the energy in the jaw. Used in conjunction with the jaw exercises, especially if the exercises are done slowly and gently, the jaw can come out of being clenched into balance and freedom.

CAREFUL EATING

Benefit: Helps to tone a double chin.

Expression: Sullen

Muscle: Temporalis

Time: Five to fifteen repetitions

Causes: The temporalis loses effectiveness when:

- thinking and perceiving are not balanced
- you act too rational when emotional
- you lack cognitive focus
- you rely on a spacey spirituality
- you hold on tightly to a preferred reality

Corrects: This exercise will:

- strengthen the relationship between thinking and perceiving
- allow a normal emotional response
- bring more energy into cognitive focus
- ground spirituality into reality

Wise application: You have too much in your head. Do Careful Eating, letting your jaw relax, and feel your mind relax. It is especially effective when done with points 1.

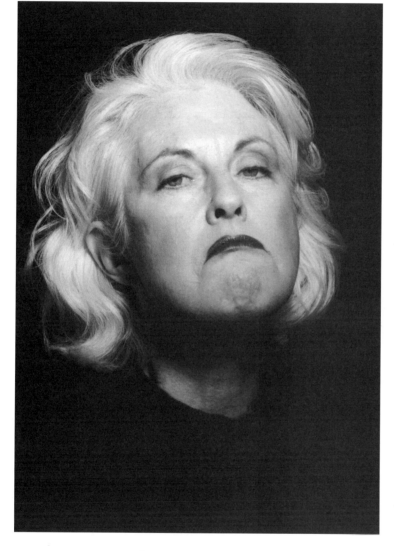

Sullen. Corners of the mouth are drawn down in a good two-year-old's pout.

1. Position your jaw and tongue.

2. Close your lips. Chew—mouth closed—stretching fully between your upper and lower teeth, with your lips firmly closed. When you chew, lower your jaw back as well as down.

3. Repeat five to fifteen times.

Acupressure points 1: Rest your fingertips lightly for one minute, or until you feel a light pulse.

Acupressure point 5: Squeeze and massage the tip of your nose and then, pressing on the tip, rotate to the right and then to the left. Pull your ears—a gentle tug on the top and the sides and finally the lobes.

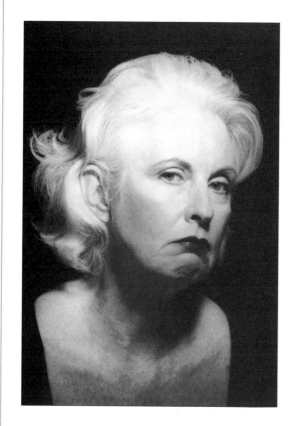

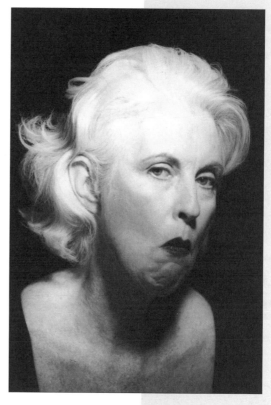

Benefit:	Helps to tone jowls and a double chin.
Expression:	Stubborn
Muscle:	Pterygoids
Time:	Five to fifteen repetitions
Causes:	This muscle loses balance when:

- your jaw is held in a forward position— anger—or in a retracted position—grief
- you take positions instead of "grinding" through a whole experience
- you hold back on your energy/aliveness
- you withhold
- you disapprove

Corrects: This exercise will:

- balance your jaw and relax the stress held there
- provide steady movement through life
- let things go
- develop a better sense of timing
- increase curiosity leading to understanding or acceptance

Wise application: When you feel too separated from life and love by your opinions, do My Way or the Highway; release the jaw back and down and hold points 7.

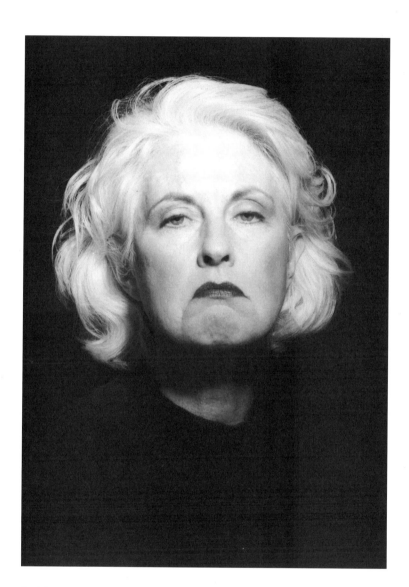

Stubborn. The jaw sets and draws back slightly.

1. Position your jaw and tongue.

2. This is an exercise to loosen your jaw. Do it slowly and gently with your jaw well positioned. Start with small circular movements. *Slowly* increase the movement as your jaw softens and opens. With your teeth slightly apart and your lips gently sealed, move your jaw back and forth and from side to side, up and down. Gently!

3. Repeat five to fifteen times.

Acupressure points 7: Touch or tap lightly.

Acupressure points 6: Press firmly, massaging in small circular motions first to your right and then to your left.

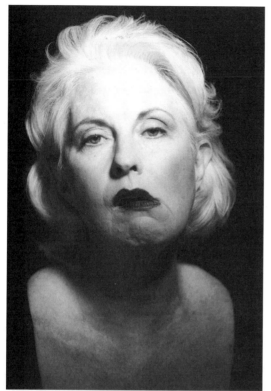

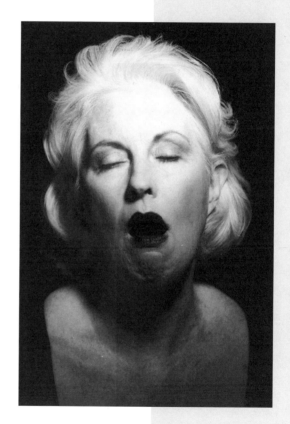

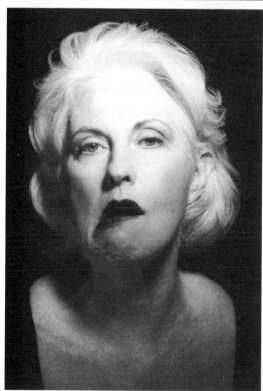

RAISE AND SMOOTH

Benefits:	Helps to firm and smooth the skin of the chin and to tone under the jaw.
Expression:	Defiant sulk
Muscle:	Mentalis
Time:	Five to fifteen repetitions
Causes:	The chin loses tone and gets squiggles from:

- inner pouting attitude
- grim determination
- dissatisfaction
- feeling isolated from old sadness and anger
- authority problems

Corrects: This exercise will:

- help you feel sweetness of heart instead of sadness
- let you feel more a part of life
- provide a sense of acceptance

Wise application: When you are feeling dissatisfied by something, doing Raise and Smooth, and then relaxing the jaw and separating your lips, may give you a new view.

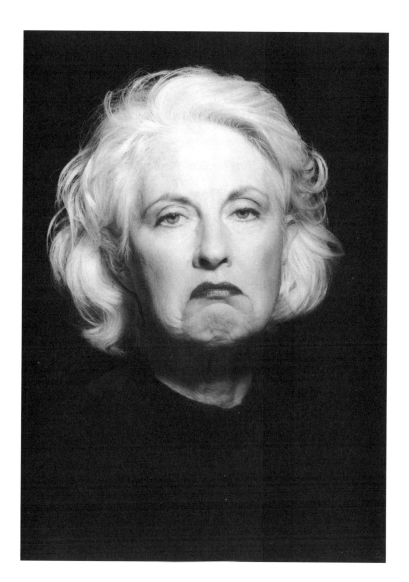

Defiant sulk. The chin pushes up, corners of the mouth go down, and the nostrils flare.

1. Position your jaw and tongue.

2. Use your chin to create a pout by pushing up with the chin muscle. Pull the chin slowly down and draw your chin back into the nonpouting position with your lips slightly separate.

3. Repeat five to fifteen times.

Acupressure points 7: Touch or tap lightly.

Acupressure points 6: Press firmly, massaging in small circular motions, first counterclockwise and then clockwise.

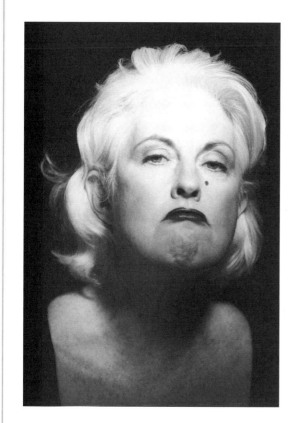

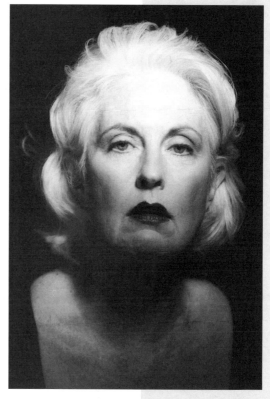

Benefit:	Helps to tone a double chin.
Expression:	You're getting a sore throat checked.
Muscles:	Digastricus, mylohyoideus
Time:	Five to fifteen repetitions
Causes:	A double chin is caused by:

- difficulty in facing and integrating life
- holding back unspoken words
- ruminating over an experience but not integrating it and moving on
- refusing to take in more experience

Corrects:	This exercise will:

- improve management of energy and stress
- ground you into reality
- develop a stronger relationship with your spiritual nature
- allow you to feel more open to taking life in, integrating it, and benefiting from it.

Wise application:	When you feel rushed, spacey, not well grounded in time and space, do Open Wide—*Ahhh* several times.

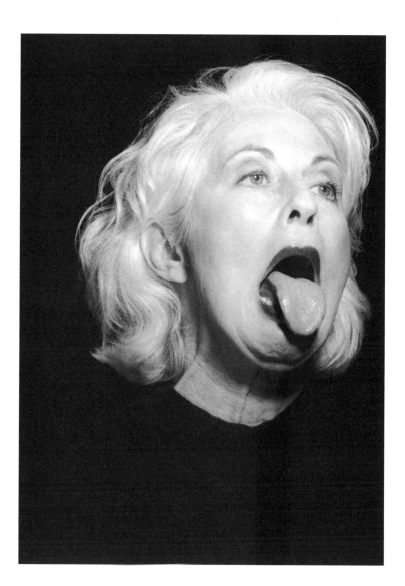

You're getting a sore throat checked. Extend the tongue out as far as you can, while your mouth opens wide.

1. Position your jaw, but positioning your tongue is not possible.

2. Drop your head back and extend your tongue out as far as you can as if to touch your chin and then your nose (this also helps to clear up a sore throat if you catch it right at the beginning). Feel the stretch deep in the throat. Return head to normal position.

3. Repeat five to fifteen times.

Acupressure points 7: Touch or tap lightly.

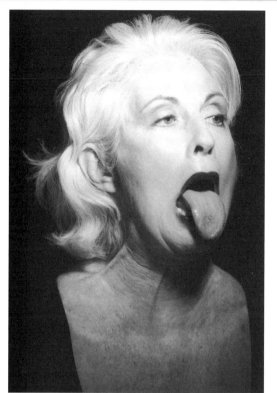

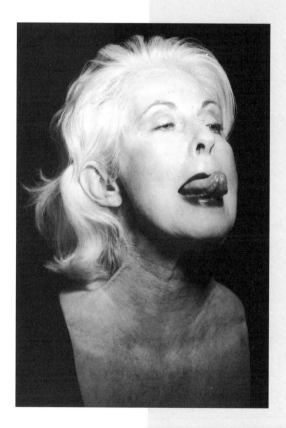

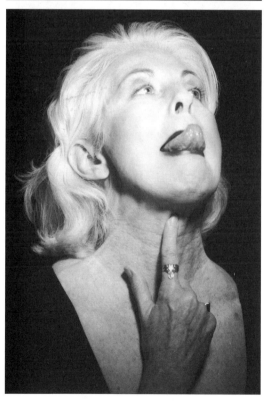

THE CALMER

Benefit:	Smooths the skin of the neck.
Expression:	Pushing down feelings by tightening the neck muscles as if to pull the head down into the neck like a turtle.
Muscle:	Platysma
Time:	Five to fifteen repetitions
Causes:	The neck wrinkles from:

- a difficulty in being able to steady energy highs and lows
- mental stress creating great tension

Corrects:	This exercise will:

- balance the highs and lows in your energy
- bring greater calm amid the haste

Wise application:	You need to settle yourself down. Do The Calmer slowly and then relax your jaw as you hold acupressure points 7.

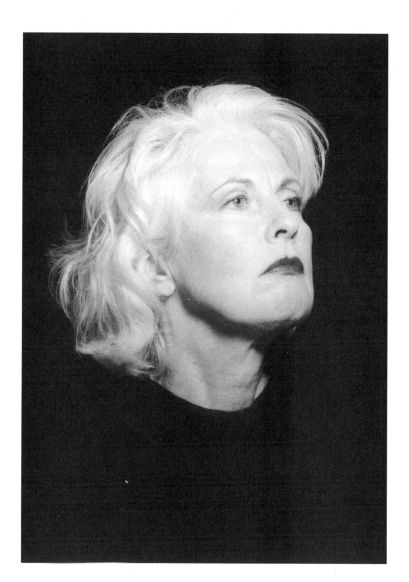

Pushing down your feelings, like a turtle pulling its head into its neck. Pull your head down into your neck and shoulders.

1. Position your jaw and tongue.

2. Drop your head back. Kiss the stars with a big smooch. Reach up with your lips, feeling the stretch down your jaw into your neck, keeping the corners of your mouth tight against your teeth. Draw your mouth into a tight grin. With your mouth in the tight grin, slowly draw your head down.

3. Repeat five to fifteen times.

   You can place your hand on your neck and feel the platysma working and smoothing the skin.

Acupressure points 7: Touch or tap lightly.

Acupressure point 5: Squeeze and massage the tip of your nose and then, pressing on the tip, rotate to the right and then to the left.

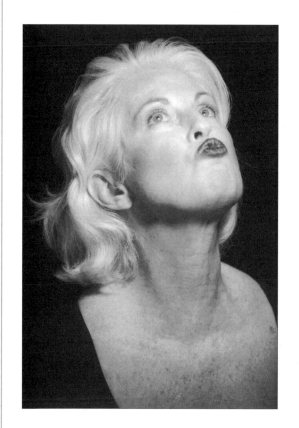

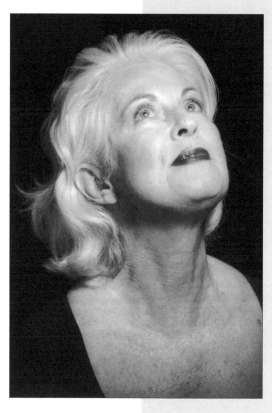

GET OUT OF MY FACE

Benefits:	Smooths the neck skin and tones under the jaw.
Expression:	Belligerent
Muscles:	All muscles of the neck
Time:	Five to fifteen repetitions
Causes:	The neck loses tone from:

- lack of groundedness
- difficulty orienting into experience
- losing one's head
- feeling unsafe

Corrects: This exercise will:

- bring a sense of standing your ground confidently and solidly
- let you know your opinions and ideas
- help you keep your head
- let you express excitement evenly

Wise application: You need to get centered, pull yourself together, and get grounded. Get Out of My Face will help.

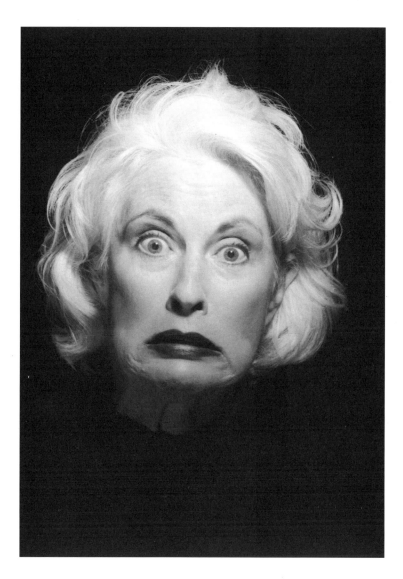

Belligerent. Tighten the jaw, neck, and lower lip muscles by contracting them down. Growl or be mad.

1. Position your jaw and tongue.

2. Make an "animal growl" look. Your lower lip may curl down. (Even making growling stay-away sounds helps.) Drop your head back so you are looking up. Using the muscles of your neck and jaw, pull your head upright. You will feel the muscles working under your jaw and down into your neck, maintaining this "growl" as you do your repetitions.

3. Repeat five to fifteen times.

Acupressure points 7: Touch or tap lightly.

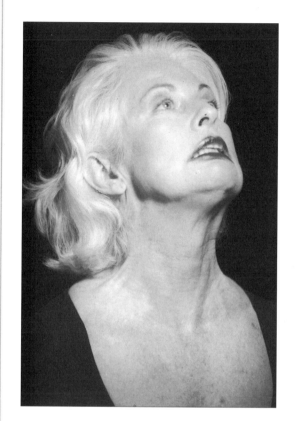

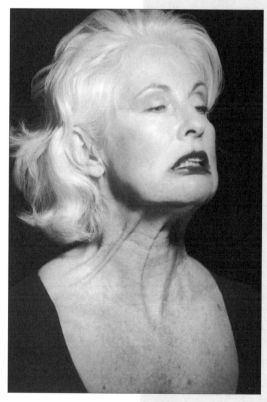

Author's Note

This is my program to create your own fresh and present Timeless Face. I hope you find personal benefit in making it your program, too. I would love to hear of your progress. My E-mail address is elinwood@aol.com. Unfortunately, my busy life may prevent me from answering everyone, but I would love to hear from you nonetheless. Which exercises do you like or dislike? Why? How has the program worked for you overall? Please feel free to keep me informed!

Best wishes,
Ellae